Obesity Discrimination

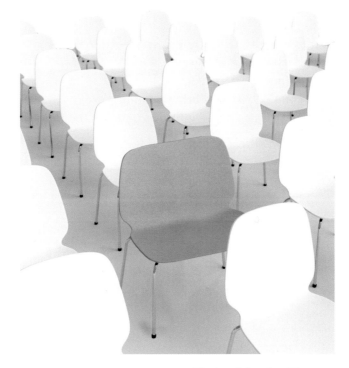

Dale-Marie Bryan

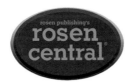

rosen publishing's
rosen
central®

New York

Published in 2009 by The Rosen Publishing Group, Inc.
29 East 21st Street, New York, NY 10010

Copyright © 2009 by The Rosen Publishing Group, Inc.

First Edition

Library of Congress Cataloging-in-Publication Data

Bryan, Dale-Marie, 1953–
Obesity discrimination / Dale-Marie Bryan.—1st ed.
    p. cm.—(Understanding obesity)
Includes bibliographical references.
ISBN-13: 978-1-4042-1766-9 (library binding)
1. Discrimination against overweight persons. 2. Obesity—Social aspects. I. Title.
RC628.B79 2009
362.196'398—dc22

2007050675

Manufactured in the United States of America

Contents

Introduction

You and your mother are comparing class photos. She shows you hers and you both laugh at her less-than-stylish outfit. But she was cool in her day. And you don't look too bad yourself. Your hair turned out nicely for once and you've definitely got her smile. But you notice a difference. The camera wasn't as kind to everyone. Is it your imagination, or are there more kids with double chins in your photo than in hers?

Health experts say there are. They are concerned about America's growing weight problem. They are so worried, in fact, that they are calling it an epidemic. An epidemic is a disease that spreads quickly and affects many, maybe millions, of people.

According to the Centers for Disease Control and Prevention (CDC), in 2003–2004, 66 million adults and 12.5 million children and teenagers were overweight or obese. That means more than four times as many kids are obese now than when your mother was your age. And it is predicted that by 2010, that number will climb to one in two young people between the ages of three and eighteen.

Whether it affects adults or young people, obesity can make life painful for those who suffer from it. They can develop serious health conditions such as heart disease, diabetes, stroke, some kinds of cancer, and gall bladder disease. They may develop mental problems like depression, which can sometimes lead to suicide. Also, attempts to deal with weight may create further problems, such as the eating disorders bulimia and anorexia.

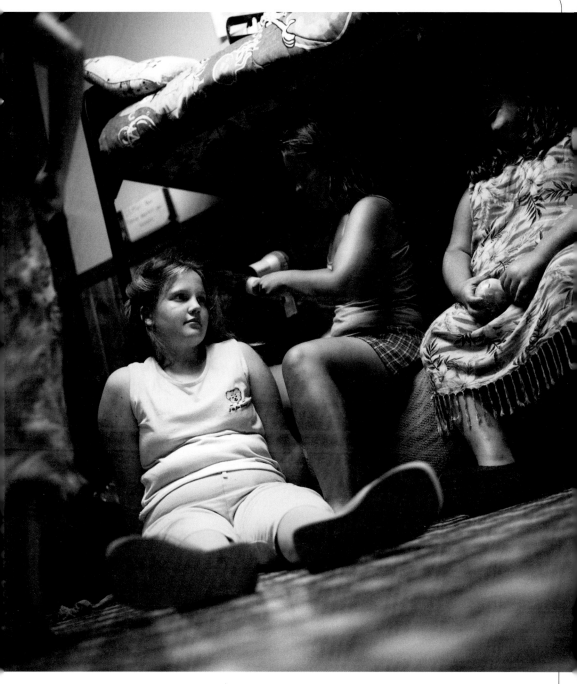

Girls attend a weight-loss camp to mold themselves into society's ideal. Many will lose weight. Some may regain it after camp.

The obese suffer emotionally as well. One of the main reasons for this is society's warped view of body size. From all sides, we hear about what a "perfect" body should be. We idolize that body and may look down on those who don't have it. We play into media and advertising messages telling us how we should look and what to do about it if we don't. We try hard to shape our bodies to fit the media mold.

This focus on the so-called ideal body can lead us to resent those we think aren't trying hard enough to achieve one. Maybe they are lazy or don't care as much as we do. This resentment can build into bias or prejudice that, in its extreme form, is hatred.

Prejudice could be considered a disease of intolerance. It causes people to discriminate against others. The latest targets of discrimination are the obese.

Chapter 1

What Is Obesity?

You've probably heard a lot of terms describing a person with a larger-than-average body size. Phrases like "too fat," "plus-sized," and "big-boned" are common. But just as there are many body sizes, there are different ideas of what a healthy weight should be. Even experts argue about how to tell.

For years, people went by charts made by Metropolitan Life, an insurance company. The figures were based on the average weights of their customers. But the charts were very limited. They didn't account for how active a person was, or, that as people aged, they naturally gained weight. The company adjusted the charts, but they still didn't give people a true picture.

Then health experts created standards, or a set of guidelines. They decided what weights would be normal, overweight, or obese. They based the standards on a special

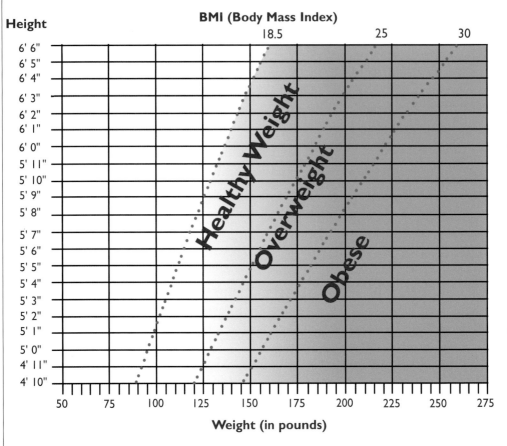

Height

BMI (Body Mass Index)

18.5   25   30

6' 6"
6' 5"
6' 4"
6' 3"
6' 2"
6' 1"
6' 0"
5' 11"
5' 10"
5' 9"
5' 8"
5' 7"
5' 6"
5' 5"
5' 4"
5' 3"
5' 2"
5' 1"
5' 0"
4' 11"
4' 10"

Healthy Weight

Overweight

Obese

50   75   100   125   150   175   200   225   250   275

Weight (in pounds)

The body mass index (BMI) became the government-approved scale for weight in 1998. Many people who ranked as having healthy weight by previous standards were considered overweight according to the BMI.

scale called the body mass index, or BMI. The BMI compares a person's height to his or her weight.

Some experts argue the BMI is still not right for everyone. They say it doesn't allow for people who weigh more because of bone structure or their amount of muscle. A fit person, like an athlete, for example, may be overweight according to the BMI.

But their extra weight comes from muscle, which weighs more than fat.

The BMI also has to be used differently for children and teenagers to allow for their growth. There are different scales for boys and girls because they grow at different rates. Their heights and weights are compared with others of their same sex and age.

Another way to judge a healthy size is to see if a person weighs more than the limits that his or her frame or skeleton should carry. This can be determined by measuring the size of the wrist and the width of the elbow.

OVERWEIGHT OR OBESE?

According to the U.S. Department of Health and Human Services, the terms "overweight" and "obese" do not mean the same thing. The term "overweight" means having "an excess of body weight compared to set standards. This may come from muscle, bone, fat, and/or body water." Obesity, however, specifically means having too much body fat.

People disagree about calling obesity a disease. Government offices like the Internal Revenue Service and the Social Security Administration classify it as one. This makes it possible for people to get governmental help with the expenses of obesity.

Others don't want to use the words "overweight" and "obese" at all because they make people link excess weight with illness. And saying all people are sick because they are over-weight isn't necessarily true, or so says Marilyn Wann, author of the book *Fat! So?* and a leader for size acceptance. She goes on to explain that the person who says fat people are sick is really

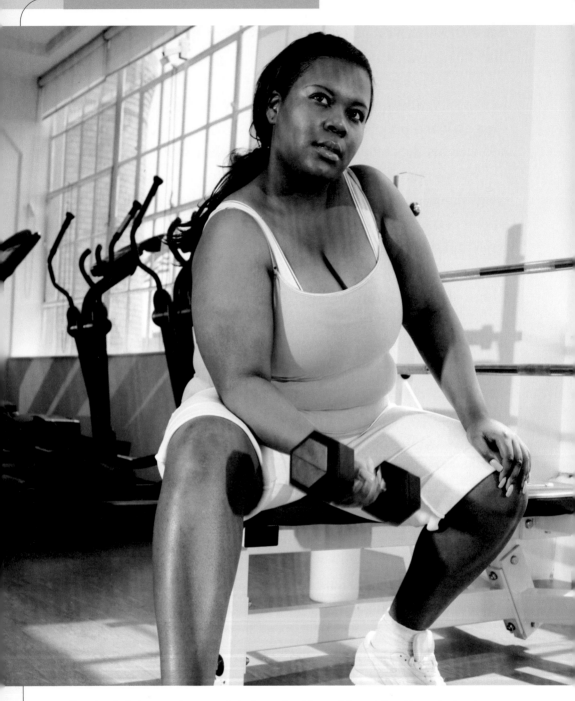

People of all sizes can improve their fitness level by weight training. Also called resistance training, weight training builds lean muscle and increases metabolism.

just lumping them together rather than trying to see them as valuable individuals.

Still others say the obesity issue is not as serious as health officials claim. Paul Campos, author of *The Obesity Myth*, says Americans are only 15 pounds (6.8 kilograms) heavier than twenty years ago. He says it is the health standards that have changed to become stricter.

No matter whom you listen to, it is important to remember that a person's size does not necessarily determine how fit he or she is. Many people exercise regularly and eat healthy diets yet still weigh more than health officials claim they should. They are fat but also fit, and not necessarily in any more danger of getting sick than the average person. Likewise, people can be thin and unfit because they are not active and do not eat well. Health should be determined more on whether a person is leading an active, body-positive lifestyle than on what a bathroom scale says. If it is caused by excessive fat, excess weight can lead to health problems, but not necessarily if it is because of higher-than-average muscle mass. It is just as important to remember that thinness or losing weight will not necessarily make a person healthier.

What Causes Obesity?

According to the Obesity Action Coalition, obesity is caused from people "taking in more calories than they burn over an extended period of time. These extra calories are stored as fat." This comes from three main things: behavior; environment, or the world around us; and family traits.

Kelly Brownell, an expert on obesity from Yale University, says we have created "a toxic environment." Toxic means

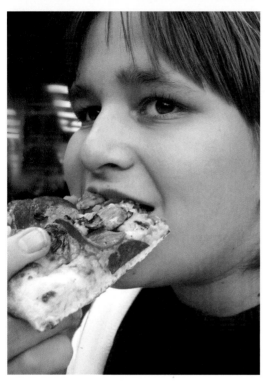

In 2004, according to the *San Francisco Chronicle*, pizza was the fourth-largest calorie contributor to American diets. In 2006, the *St. Paul Pioneer Press* stated Americans averaged 46 slices yearly.

harmful, destructive, or deadly. Brownell believes people today are exposed to high-calorie, high-fat, highly advertised foods that are cheap and easy to get. She says that, combined with a lifestyle where we are not as physically active, has led to the increase in obesity.

Our way of life does have a lot to do with how our bodies react to food. Today's families are on the go. They pick up fast-food meals to eat in their cars on the way to soccer practice, dance lessons, or school activities. And fast-food places make it cheaper to fill up hungry families by offering super-sized portions.

A report from the American Dietetic Association says eating healthy foods may cost too much for many families. With only so much to spend on food, they buy what will fill them up. Often, that is not the foods that are healthiest. The report also says families would have to spend from 43 to 70 cents of every dollar to buy the amount of fresh fruits and vegetables they are supposed to have. That's OK for higher-income families. But poor families might not be able to do it. If they get government help like food stamps, they can only use them for certain types of food. Many of those are more processed foods that last longer and are easier to provide. While such foods may be convenient, fast, and filling, they also contain more fat and sugar. So, what people save in time and money, they pay for in vitamins, minerals, and other nutrients.

Also, people don't have to put in long hours of physical labor to provide for their families. In the past, most families worked on or earned a living from farming. They spent long hours raising food for themselves and for others. It was hard work but good exercise. People didn't need to get on a treadmill to burn off Mom's apple pie or fried chicken. They just hoed crops, hauled water, or chopped wood. Now, according to the U.S. Department of Agriculture (USDA), only 2 percent of the nation's population earns a living from farms or ranches.

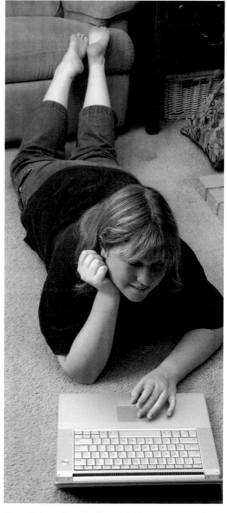

The Kaiser Family Foundation reports that American teens use media for about five-and-a-half hours a day. Exercising for one of those hours would meet the USDA's recommended allowance.

Labor-saving devices have made life easier. They give us more free time to spend watching television or e-mailing friends. We drive rather than walk to most places. Because neighborhoods aren't safe, children don't play outside or walk to and from school like they used to.

Families no longer eat and play together as much. Instead, the parents are working to make ends meet while the children wait for them to return home. Their only companions are television, computer and video games, and snacks.

MEAN GENES

Cruel as it may seem, your size may also depend on your heredity, or the characteristics you get from your ancestors. If you see a child who is overweight, chances are that one or both of his or her parents are overweight and were as youngsters, too. Studies show overweight children have a 70 percent chance of being overweight adults. But this doesn't necessarily mean an overweight family overeats. According to various studies, it is likely they share a gene that makes it easier to convert food to fat.

For thousands of years, this was a good thing. People who shared this gene were more likely to live through times when they were not able to grow or find enough food. These people survived to pass these "stronger" genes from generation to generation. Today, though, with food so plentiful and easy to get, these fat storage genes curse us. Whatever food we take in is ours to keep around our hips, thighs, and stomachs. What was once a life-saving trait is now a life-threatening plague.

Michael Pollan, in his book *The Omnivore's Dilemma*, believes that we, as omnivores, have to make many food choices because our bodies need many different nutrients. (Omnivores are animals that eat both plants and other animals.) Pollan writes, "Our taste buds help . . . [steer] us toward sweetness."

Beverly J. Cowart, an expert on senses, agrees. She says animals use their sense of taste to decide what to eat. "Many poisonous or indigestible plants are bitter; fruit . . . is sweet; and salt, necessary for human survival, is appealing." So, if you hear someone say they were born with a sweet tooth, they may be right.

According to C. Ronald Kahn and Mary Iacocca, German researchers and professors of medicine at Harvard Medical School, another gene called PPAR controls the amount and size of fat cells. They get stuck, they say, in the "on" position, "and these cells get fatter faster than normal fat cells." Kahn and Iacocca are continuing to study this mutation but think it may be part of the obesity problem for some people.

According to a recent study by Dr. Brian Morris and his colleagues at the University of Sydney in Australia, another gene they call Ser363 may cause obesity, too. "All study participants who had two copies of the gene, one from each parent, were overweight. So were [most] people who had just one copy of the gene." The researchers think the Ser363 gene causes a person's body to be more sensitive to hormones that have a main role in fat and protein metabolism, or the way a body uses energy, and where fat is distributed on the body.

Other researchers at Washington University in St. Louis, Missouri, studied fat and thin mice and found a bacteria in the gut that makes putting on fat easier. Researchers Jeffrey Gordon and Ruth Ley found similar bacteria in humans. These bacteria have a hormone that makes them really good at taking calories from food. Gordon and Ley think this may have something to do with the reason some people are more likely to gain weight than others.

We can't escape the fact that our bodies have been conditioned over millions of years to look for sweet and salty foods. We also can't help what genes and bacteria in our gut cause our bodies to do. Scientists will continue to look for information that may help us understand why our bodies react to food the way they do. Yet, some, like Dr. Ali Mokdad of the CDC, say, "We believe the culprits are still lack of exercise and increased consumption."

Chapter 2

What's the Big Deal?

"So?" you might say. "I'm not overweight or obese. Why should I care?" One reason is because even if you aren't, more than half the U.S. population is. So, it's likely friends or family members—people you care about—are worrying about their weight. If they don't eat a healthy diet and get enough exercise, they may have a reason to worry. According to health experts, overweight and obese people run a much greater risk of developing serious illnesses like heart disease, high blood pressure, and some kinds of cancer. They may also get a disease called diabetes, which starts when glucose, a kind of sugar, builds up in the blood. These illnesses claim thousands of lives each year.

Another reason to care is because people fighting weight issues sometimes feel bad about themselves. They may suffer from depression. Depression causes people

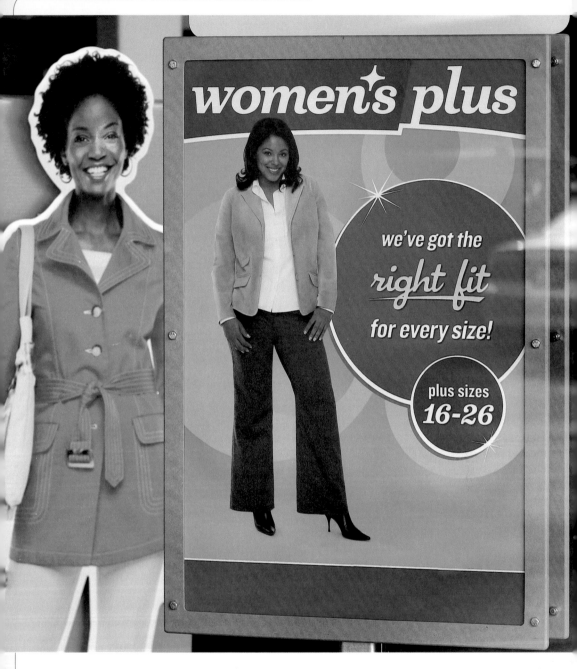

With an increase in the number of overweight people in the United States, some stores have expanded their plus-sized line of clothing.

to lose interest in the world around them. They may not be able to work, or they may be angry or unable to show love and affection. Living with these conditions is hard on everyone.

But it is easy to understand why some fat people become depressed. The media, including television, movies, magazines, and books, spread the idea that thin is "in" and fat is "bad." As larger-sized people hear these constant messages, they may come to believe them. They may begin to hate their bodies. Some even have thoughts of suicide.

No matter what your BMI, you face weight issues every day. Whether it's worry over a family member's weight-related illness, your friends' constant talk of dieting, or remarks and jokes people make at school or in the media, information about overweight and obesity surround you. And it's pretty scary stuff. But it is how you react to weight issues that makes the difference, and learning all you can is the first step.

DISCRIMINATION: AN UGLY WORD

Even though you may not think so, when one person makes fun of another, it is a form of discrimination according to the Council on Size and Weight Discrimination.

"What?" you ask. "I thought discrimination was when people couldn't drink at the same water fountains or didn't have ramps to get in and out of places." While that's true, and people have suffered throughout history, discrimination hasn't gone away. It's still common and just as ugly today.

Discrimination is the act of treating someone differently because of a dislike or hatred for that person's group, race, or religion. A related word, "bias," describes the favoring of one group over another based on cloudy or false judgments. An example would be the members of a chess club barring girls from joining because they say girls aren't good at strategy games.

Prejudices are the feelings and opinions behind discrimination and bias. When a person is prejudiced, it means he or she is prejudging people because of the religion, race, nationality, or group they belong to. Prejudices are strong and hard to change. They are often rooted in fear and ignorance. You would be displaying your prejudices if you didn't want certain kids sitting with you at lunch because they weren't good at sports or spoke a different language.

People often base their prejudices on stereotypes. Stereotypes describe a whole group of people in a specific way. Such descriptions lump people together and tag them with a trait, which is usually negative. Even a comment that is supposed to be a compliment can be a stereotype and hurtful.

How Do People Become Prejudiced?

Children imitate the actions of their families. Even if their families work toward not showing bias, children see and hear it in the media or from others around them. The more children are exposed to biased talk and actions, the more likely they are to view those negative ways of thinking and acting as "normal." They may see one group as not being as good as another and think they deserve to be treated badly. Unless someone teaches them differently, children will carry these beliefs into their adult lives.

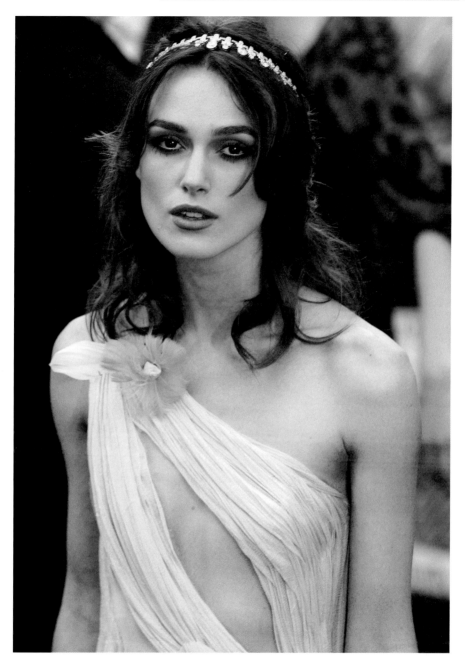

Young people often try to imitate their favorite celebrities, like Keira Knightley. However, some celebrities are unhealthily thin and may prove to be dangerous role models.

Myths and Facts

Myth: **Overweight people eat more than thin people.**
Fact: Studies have shown that some overweight people eat similarly or sometimes less than thin people. Many eat less often or skip meals.

Myth: **Fat people are lazy.**
Fact: A person's size has no relation to how well or hard he or she works or to what that person would like to do with his or her life. Fat students are just as likely to get top grades as thin students. The fact that they may not be as active in sports may have more to do with how other people treat them and their negative feelings about their bodies rather than laziness.

Myth: **Overweight people have no self-control.**
Fact: It takes a lot of self-control to deal with the teasing and ridicule that fat people hear every day. Also, many stick with diets to lose hundreds of pounds, only to have the weight come back. But this is due to the way their bodies use and retain energy rather than a lack of willpower. One obese woman observed that she quit smoking after thirty years. If that didn't show willpower, she didn't know what did.

Myth: **Children don't worry about their weight.**
Fact: According to the Council on Size and Weight Discrimination, 42 percent of first-, second-, and third-grade girls want to lose weight, and 45 percent of boys and girls in grades three through six said they were sometimes or often on diets.

Myth: **Every U.S. state has a law that protects obese people from discrimination.**
Fact: Michigan is the only U.S. state that has laws on the books that make weight discrimination illegal.

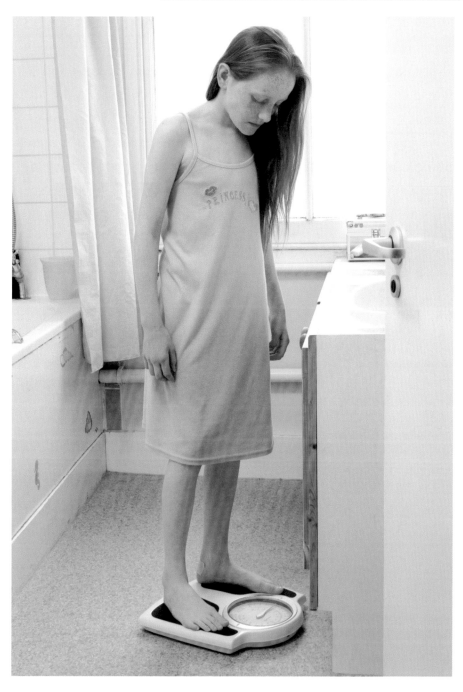

When young people measure their self-worth against what they think of as "the perfect body," they may undervalue their own beauty, talents, and interests.

THE OBESE: THE LATEST VICTIMS

Every day, people of all ages face discrimination like this and worse because of their size or appearance. According to the Obesity Action Coalition, 63 percent of girls and 58 percent of boys report being teased or bullied by others their age. Of these, 30 percent of girls and 24 percent of boys are teased because of their weight. In the *Journal of American Medicine*, some obese students rated their lives as being as bad as those of children with cancer.

Whom Does Obesity Discrimination Hurt?

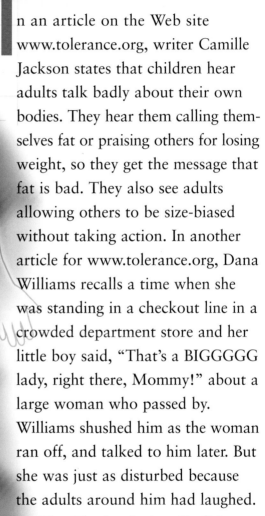

In an article on the Web site www.tolerance.org, writer Camille Jackson states that children hear adults talk badly about their own bodies. They hear them calling themselves fat or praising others for losing weight, so they get the message that fat is bad. They also see adults allowing others to be size-biased without taking action. In another article for www.tolerance.org, Dana Williams recalls a time when she was standing in a checkout line in a crowded department store and her little boy said, "That's a BIGGGGG lady, right there, Mommy!" about a large woman who passed by. Williams shushed him as the woman ran off, and talked to him later. But she was just as disturbed because the adults around him had laughed.

The Obesity Action Coalition agrees that obese people are blamed for being overweight. Many people believe they are fat because

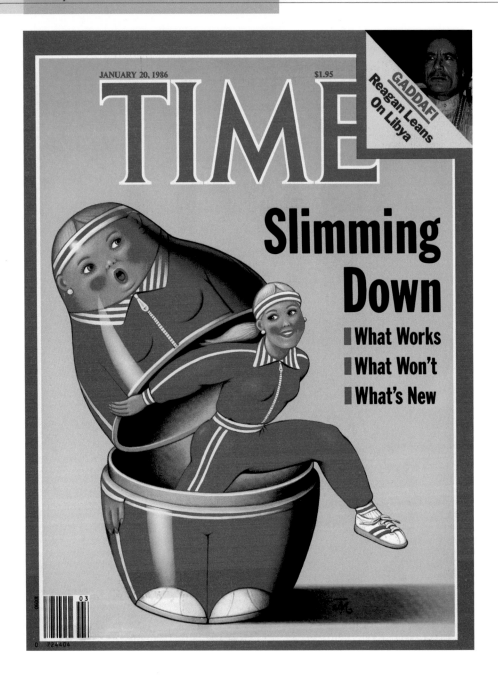

Society's preoccupation with appearance and body image has created an atmosphere where many feel that if they aren't dieting, they aren't normal.

they just aren't trying hard enough. There is no sympathy for those they think can't control themselves. Yet, if they believe the person's weight problem comes from something they can't help, such as a medical condition like thyroid disease, they are more understanding.

People also learn to be biased from messages in the media. In the days before television and movies, people who were heavier were thought to be healthier. During hard times like the Depression in the 1920s, more weight was a sign of wealth, too. If you had enough money to buy enough food to get fat, you were pretty well off. Fat babies were a source of pride because they showed the family was being well taken care of. In later years, curvy women like Marilyn Monroe and Jane Russell became popular. Over the last fifty years, however, people's ideas shifted. Fat was no longer good. Thin was in.

Jean Rubel, Ph.D., founder of Anorexia Nervosa and Related Eating Disorders, Inc., wrote about this change in an article for *Radiance* magazine: "Look at the world young people live in. Think of your favorite television show or movie. There are probably more thin characters than fat ones and the thin ones are . . . popular, beautiful, powerful, and successful. Fat people, if there are any, are probably . . . evil, weak, stupid, silly, or [greedy]. Now . . . would a child want to be fat or thin?"

A 2002 study published in *Research and Practice* by Greenberg, Eastin, Hofschire, Brownell and Lachian, showed that, in real life, one in four women is obese, but on television only three out of every one hundred women are portrayed as heavier. It also showed that men in real life are three times more likely to be large-sized than the men on television.

Advertising makes the problem worse. A study by Philip N. Myers and Frank A. Biocca found that in 4,294 network television commercials, 1 out of every 3.8 showed some kind of message telling viewers what is attractive and what is not. Another study, by Alfreiter, Elzinga, and Gordon, found the average teenager sees about 5,000 "attractiveness" commercials a year.

Mass media magazines add to the problem. According to researchers Guillen and Barr, over a twenty-year-study of one teen magazine, 74 percent of the fitness and health articles told readers that the reason to start exercising was "to be more attractive." Another 51 percent stated "to lose weight or burn calories" was the reason for exercise.

The fashion industry plays a part in what people believe, too. The average model is 5'9" tall and weighs 110 pounds (49.8 kg). Yet, the average woman is 5'4" and weighs 147 pounds (66.6 kg). A study at the University of Missouri–Columbia found that after three minutes of looking at fashion magazines, women felt less satisfied with their bodies. "It had been thought that women who are heavier feel worse than a thinner woman after viewing pictures of [women thought to be] ideal in the mass media. The study results do not support that theory," says Laurie Mintz, associate professor of education, school, and counseling psychology in the MU College of Education. "Weight was not a factor. Viewing these pictures was just bad for everyone."

It is no wonder that these constant messages on television, in movies, and in magazines influence how we look at each other and have made us size-biased.

"It's only a little teasing," you may say. "The guys kid me about stuff all the time. They're just having a good time. Get over it!" An article by Dorothea Ross, Ph.D., and S. Ross, Ph.D.,

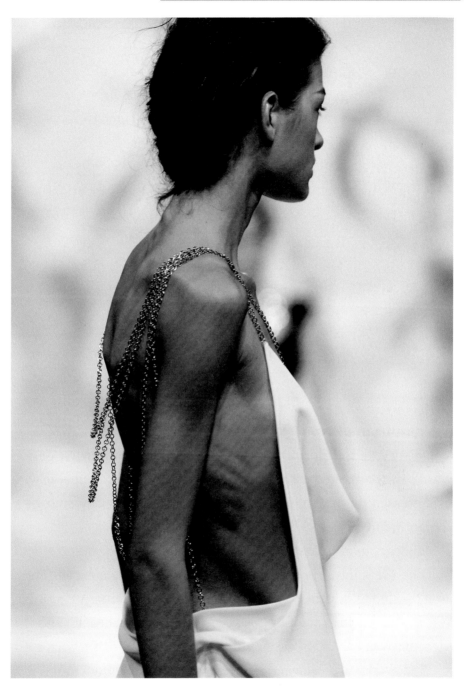

Some fashion models have literally starved themselves for their jobs. In recent years, this has driven the fashion industry to rethink its weight requirements.

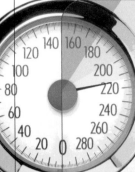

Facts About Facing Obesity

1. If Barbie were a real person, she would be 7'2" tall and weigh 101 pounds.
2. One-third of American women wear size 16 or larger.
3. Seventy percent of normal-weight girls in high school feel fat and are on a diet.
4. Forty-five percent of boys and girls in third through sixth grade want to be thinner.
5. Forty-six percent of nine- to eleven-year-old girls have dieted.
6. During puberty, girls' bodies tend to gain ten inches in height and 40 to 50 pounds (18 to 22 kg).

in a nursing publication says that teasing is rarely innocent fun. When surveyed, children who had leukemia said the worst part wasn't the pain, or the chemo, or the possibility of dying—it was being teased by other children for not having hair as a result of chemotherapy.

Students in all parts of the country suffer teasing, ridicule, and bullying every day. They sit by themselves. They are ignored. They aren't included in games and activities. Sometimes they are abused. When students hear the phrases "the fight against obesity" and the "war on weight" in the media, they make targets of the victims.

Those who aren't overweight can't understand how much it hurts, Frances Berg, a nutritionist and weight authority from North Dakota, says.

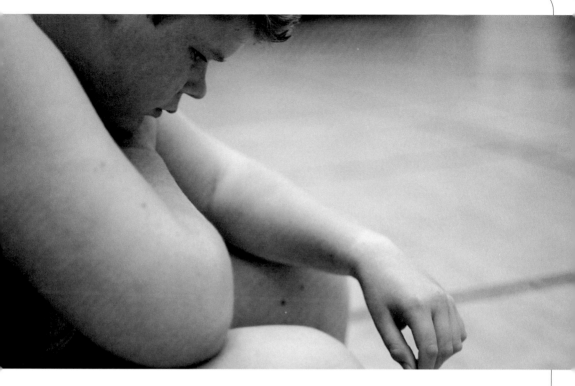

The media often glamorize a muscular male physique. This can make overweight boys dissatisfied with their bodies. Some develop eating disorders or use steroids in an effort to conform.

Michael Loewy, a psychology professor from the University of North Dakota, agrees. "It is amazing that so many fat children survive [being teenagers], given the hatred and meanness directed at them." Students from everywhere tell the stories.

DISCRIMINATE? WHO ME?

Nearly everyone is guilty of having stereotyped an overweight person at least once. Many times, it's children or teens with low self-esteem or who have suffered the effects of weight discrimination themselves who do the teasing. Perhaps they want to make themselves feel better by picking on someone they see as being worse off than they are. Maybe they are trying to fit in. Maybe they hope if they tease, they won't be teased themselves.

Teachers and school officials discriminate against obese students, too. A teacher may make comments or suggestions that make fat children feel bad about their bodies. They may exclude the students from activities because of their size. They may grade them differently because of their feelings about their own weight. They may ignore it when others students torment fat students, thinking they deserve it, or, if they hear the "truth," they might do something about it.

Discrimination happens in families as well. A fat child often becomes the scapegoat, or the reason for everyone's problems in a family. Brothers and sisters, even parents, blame the child and his or her fatness for everything from a father not getting a promotion to siblings not making the "right" friends.

Parents may favor the thin sibling, giving him or her more support and privileges than the fat child. At home, the fat child's life revolves around weight and eating habits. Meal times and outings become painful with family members watching every mouthful.

The media discriminate on television, in books and magazines, and even on billboards. In a recent press release, the National Association to Advance Fat Acceptance (NAAFA) demanded that Metro West Community Health Care Foundation in Massachusetts stop its ad campaign on the radio, on television, and in print against childhood obesity. It said the foundation must also take

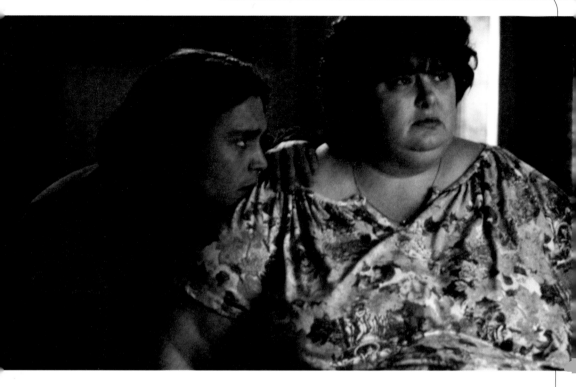

Darlene Cates played Johnny Depp's obese mother in the movie *What's Eating Gilbert Grape?* Cates was discovered on a talk show about people too heavy to leave the house.

down its billboards showing fat kids. The parents, who are fighting traffic, won't see the signs, but their obese children will. "Their campaign against fat children . . . promotes fear and hatred of larger bodies and body obsession in children [that may lead to] eating disorders."

DISCRIMINATION TEST

OK, so you don't call fat people names or make rude comments around them. But could you still be prejudiced? Ask yourself these questions to find out:

1. Do you talk about others' weight?
2. Do you make an effort to include or make friends with kids of different shapes and sizes?
3. Do you talk about diets, read nutrition labels, or make health comments in front of a large person, hoping he or she will take the hint?
4. When a teacher divides your class into teams, do you get mad if a fat kid is on yours?
5. Do you stand by or laugh when your friends tease people with differences?
6. Do you make excuses to get out of going places with your parents or family members who are fat?
7. Do you think it is nicer to ignore fat kids rather than talk to them?

Obesity is a hot topic on television, in movies, in books, and in magazines. People who are not fat cannot understand what it's like, yet many are curious about it. Rather than involving fat people themselves, the media has thin actors wear fat suits to "experience" being fat. People learn different things from the experience.

For her talk show, supermodel Tyra Banks wore a fat suit for fifteen hours. She was in a store, on a bus, and on three blind dates. "The people were staring and laughing in my face . . . that shocked me the most," she said. "As soon as I entered the store . . . when I went shopping . . . I immediately heard snickers . . . I was appalled. There's no excuse for rudeness. There's no excuse for ugliness. And there's no excuse for nastiness and that's what I experienced."

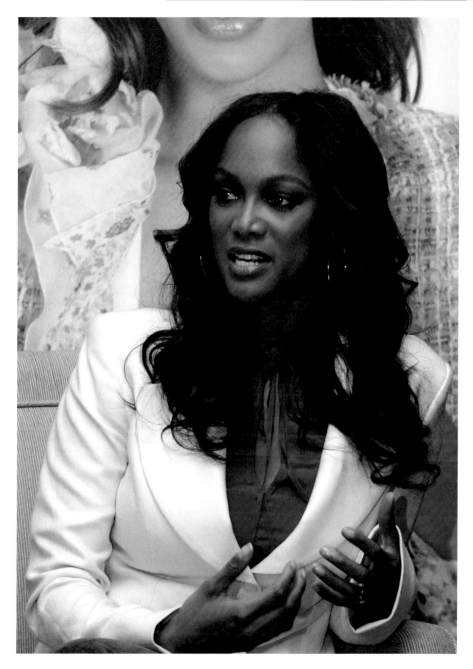

Tyra Banks spent fifteen hours in a fat suit as an experiment to test how much differently she would be perceived and treated by others.

"No one so much as even looked at me," actress Gwyneth Paltrow said of walking through a hotel lobby in her fat suit for the movie *Shallow Hal*. "It was terribly isolating."

In a 1993 *Ladies' Home Journal* article, Leslie Lambert tells of the week she spent in a fat suit. "One morning I gained 150 pounds, and my whole life changed. . . . I became angry. Angry because what I experienced in the week that I wore a 'fat suit' . . . was that our society not only hates fat people, it feels entitled to [take part] in prejudice that at many levels [is as bad as] racism and religious [discrimination]. And in a country that prides itself on being sensitive to the handicapped and the homeless, the obese continue to be the target of . . . abuse [by our culture]."

Rebecca Puhl, of the Rudd Center for Food Policy and Obesity, says that wearing fat suits can have a bad effect, too, such as when actors wear them in movies that make fun of fat people. "The idea of wearing a fat suit could be useful in cases when it's used . . . to increase awareness about weight stigma and prejudice, but the current trend is to dress up slim actors in fat suits for the . . . purpose of being a target of humor, embarrassment, and ridicule. . . . It seems to me that fat suits are mostly just reinforcing offensive stereotypes and worsening bias."

Chapter 4

Obesity Discrimination and the Law

Experiencing fat discrimination while wearing a fat suit does not touch the scope of the problem. Like bodies themselves, obesity discrimination comes in many forms and affects both young and old. Many times, it negatively shapes young people's futures. Of all places, the local health clinic or hospital is where a person should feel sure of finding help and compassion. But for the obese, that is often not true. Undersized medical gowns and too-small examination tables and equipment like MRIs and CAT scans play a part in making fat people feel uncomfortable.

DISCRIMINATION BY PROFESSIONALS

Worse than that is having to face biased doctors and nurses. According to the Obesity Action Coalition, doctors tend to blame the fat person's weight for his or her

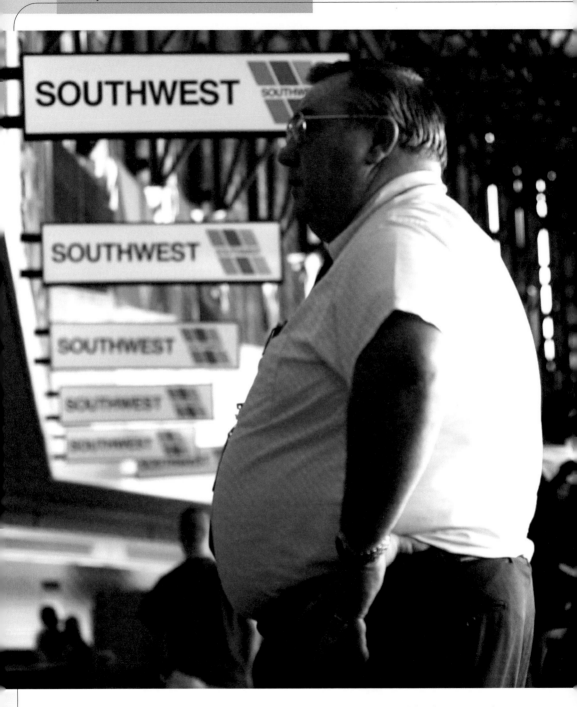

Southwest Airlines has come under attack lately over its policy requiring heavy people to pay for an extra seat if necessary.

medical conditions rather than analyzing the symptoms. Doctors spend less time with them and have less discussion. Because of this, they are not as careful about diagnosing health problems and are quick to blame overweight people for the problems. This makes the obese less likely to seek health care, which can make their medical conditions worse. They also don't get routine checkups, and they delay or cancel appointments out of fear. To make matters worse, they are often denied medical insurance or have to pay much more for it.

According to the Obesity Action Coalition, even psychologists think obese patients have more problems, worse emotional symptoms, and more negative characteristics. They also believe they are less likely to be successful with treatment.

In a study by Dr. Rebecca Puhl of the Rudd Center for Food Policy and Obesity, nurses said they viewed the obese as lazy, unsuccessful, and not willing to follow a doctor's orders. Thirty-one percent said they'd rather not take care of fat patients. Twenty-four percent said that obese patients disgusted them. Another 12 percent said they didn't want to touch obese patients.

On a trip around many major cities, a person can witness fat discrimination nearly everywhere. There are the turnstiles to subways and amusement parks that are impossible to navigate. Doorways and stairs are too narrow. People frown if the obese take up more than their share of space on elevators, in restaurants, or at social events.

DISCRIMINATION IN DAILY LIFE

Overweight people often cannot attend movies, concerts, or programs because theater seats are too small. The seats are made

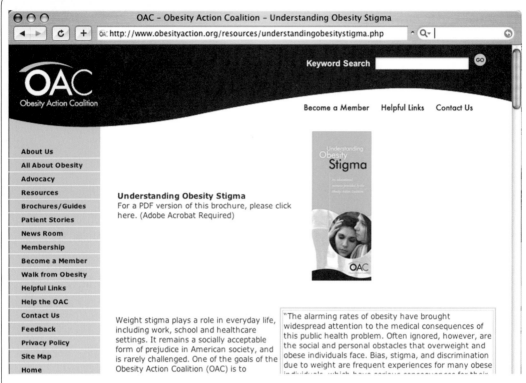

○ ○ ○   OAC – Obesity Action Coalition – Understanding Obesity Stigma

◄ ► C + OAC http://www.obesityaction.org/resources/understandingobesitystigma.php ∧ Q▾ |

The Obesity Action Coalition provides a variety of information about the obesity issue. Part of its mission is to get rid of the negative stigma that is attached to all types of obesity.

to pack in as many customers as possible, so the fat person loses out. Restroom stalls and toilets are made for smaller frames, too, as are seats on amusement park rides, trains, and buses. According to Susannah Bryan in an article for the *South Florida Sun-Sentinel*, airlines are known for poor treatment of the obese. Or, obese people are made to pay for two or more seats. "I've had ticket agents ask me if I want to buy a second seat. It's embarrassing. It's another situation where fat people are treated . . . unfairly," says Bettye Travis, a spokeswoman for the National Association to Advance Fat Acceptance. "We don't fit in the seats. The [bathrooms] are almost impossible. The week before I fly it's not fear of flying, it's fear of fitting that gets to me."

According to the Council on Size and Weight Discrimination, housing agencies, landlords, and real estate agents sometimes prevent the obese from moving into neighborhoods by not renting them apartments or houses.

In its pamphlet, *Understanding Obesity Stigma,* the Obesity Action Coalition (OAC) says obese students report not being accepted into the universities they wanted and that they were dismissed from college for being overweight They also say obese students' parents are not as likely to help them with college expenses. Professors, too, let their biases against students' weight affect the way they grade and whether they recommend them for jobs.

When they finish school, young people who are overweight often do not get jobs they are qualified for, the OAC continues. They sometimes have to take lower-paying jobs. Bosses tend to hire them only for work where they will not be seen. They are also paid less. The OAC says obese women are paid 12 percent less than thin women doing the same job, and they are not promoted as often. In addition, the obese are less likely to get hired for higher-level jobs and are more likely to get fired due to prejudiced employers, despite good employment records.

Chapter 5

The Effects of Obesity Discrimination

besity discrimination affects people in many ways. In an effort to stop the teasing and ridicule, many turn to dieting. Researchers say that every year, Americans spend between $6 billion and $50 billion on managing their weight. Yet, statistics show that diets don't work.

Dieting can lead to health problems, particularly if the dieter is not yet fully grown. It can also cause imbalances in the way the body uses food, making weight gain easier. Dieting can be dangerous, too, especially if it leads to eating disorders such as anorexia and bulimia.

Anorexia is a disease in which people starve themselves, yet still see themselves as fat. Bulimics binge on huge amounts of food, then get rid of it by making themselves throw up. The death rate for these diseases is between 5 and 20 percent, according to the *American Journal of Psychiatry*.

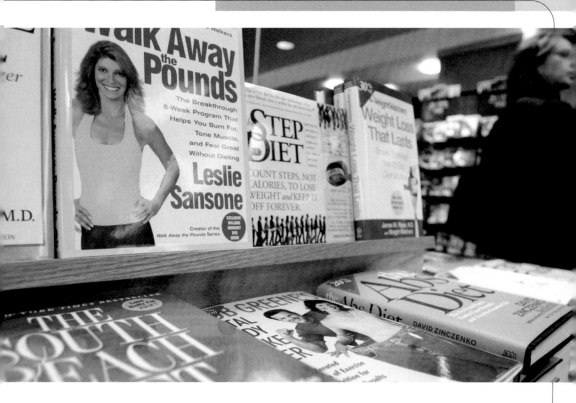

Diet books of every type crowd bookstore shelves. Rather than promoting healthy eating and physical fitness, however, many of these books focus primarily on weight loss, regardless of a person's health.

WHAT ARE PEOPLE DOING ABOUT OBESITY DISCRIMINATION?

Obesity discrimination happens when people focus more on someone's size than personality. But more people are learning to accept their own bodies and others as they are.

Speaking Out

In an article in *USA Today*, Donna Freydkin reports that in Hollywood and the fashion industry, women are beginning to appreciate their bodies instead of starve them.

Jennifer Hudson, who played Effie in *Dream Girls*, says, "I'm unique around here. I love my size and I think everybody should have some kind of meat on their bones."

Tyra Banks comments in the *USA Today* article, "I thank the Lord for Jennifer Hudson and the attention and coverage she's getting. She's curvy and beautiful. Beyoncé [Knowles], myself, all women who have curves are embracing [them] and that needs to continue."

"In Hollywood, there's always an eye on your weight," actress Eva Mendes remarks in the same article, "[but] I don't fall for that pressure."

In her Golden Globes speech, America Ferrera, star of *Ugly Betty*, said, "I hear from young girls . . . how [my character] makes them feel worthy and lovable and that they have more to offer to the world than they thought."

Carmen Marc Valvo explains. "In Hollywood, it's always been size 0 or 2 and we're starting to stray from that. Queen Latifah is a prime example. A lot of headway is being made."

Reed Krakoff, a creative coach, director, and vice president of the Council of Fashion Designers of America, says, "We've gone through a period where there has been a lot of focus on women who are too thin. There was a trend toward the very thin, and now there's a trend toward more shapely. People's perception of what's beautiful and acceptable on the red carpet is [changing], and it's great that girls can see different role models with different body types."

Accepting Ourselves

People are banning together and starting programs to help young people appreciate their bodies. The NAAFA Kids Project is one

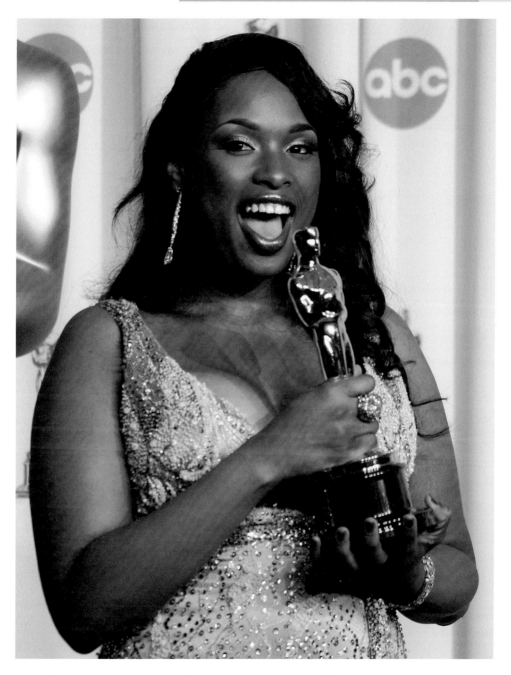

Jennifer Hudson, who won an Oscar for her portrayal of Effie in *Dream Girls*, says of her weight, "I wouldn't change myself for anything or anybody." In March 2007, she appeared on the cover of *Vogue*.

of them. NAAFA provides speakers and teaching materials on accepting your body as it is. Here are some things kids said about the talks:

- I learned that nobody has the "wrong" body size.
- I think the speaker is right, but it is hard to let go of beauty standards taught since birth.
- I learned that no matter what your body size is, if you're OK with who you are and lead a healthy lifestyle, there's nothing wrong with you.

"When I talk about body image and self-esteem, about fat and thin, I can see the relief on kids' faces," says Marilyn Wann, one of the project's speakers. "We have to break the taboo around these subjects . . . for the sake of young people, who might otherwise waste their lives and seriously damage their health in their attempts to achieve 'perfect thighs.'"

Fighting for Rights

Others are fighting for their rights, such as Jennifer Portnick of San Francisco. She wanted to be an aerobics instructor for a national health club company. But it wouldn't hire her because it said her 240-pound (108 kg) frame didn't give her a "fit appearance." The company changed its attitude, however, when she brought the case to court, saying that "it may be possible for people of [different] sizes to be fit." Portnick went on to become certified by the Aerobics and Fitness Association of America and to start her own classes. She was also hired by the East Bay YMCA.

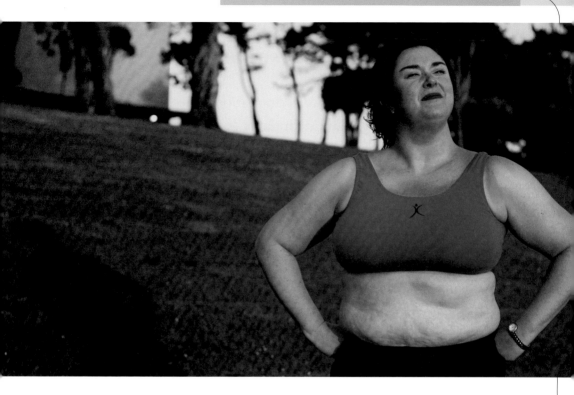

Jennifer Portnick became a certified fitness instructor, starting her own classes, despite meeting resistance because of her appearance.

Still others are writing about it. "I'm tired of all this weight-loss stuff," says Wendy Shanker, author of *The Fat Girl's Guide to Life*. "I'm tired of people pushing away bread baskets in restaurants; I'm tired of hearing women talk trash about themselves; I'm tired of being told how worthless I am because my body looks the way it does. I'm hoping to change our attitudes about this whole body image business. It is a business. It is an image. But it is YOUR body, which contains YOUR mind, which is a whole lot easier to change than the width of your thighs or the shape of your [bottom]."

Ways You Can Deal with Weight Discrimination

Whether you face weight and discrimination issues or not, there are many options for dealing with them. As with any challenge, knowing some strategies can give you an edge.

1. **Be prepared.** Make up a top-ten list of great things about you and write it on a note card. Repeat the list hourly until you know it by heart. Or, put the card in your pocket or use it as a bookmark. Whenever rude remarks come your way, take out your card and repeat your list to yourself. Remind yourself that you are a worthy and beautiful person. Negative comments are only as powerful as you allow them to be.

2. **Find your game face.** Practice your smile. Prejudiced people expect their comments to hurt, and they relish seeing the pain they cause. Smiling at them deprives them of their fun. If you feel like crying, try to wait until they can't see you. Also, improve your body language. Hold your head up and shoulders back. Walk with purpose. Look like you mean business. It's harder to pick on a person who looks strong.

3. **Choose your stones.** Remember that old saying "Sticks and stones may break my bones but words can never hurt me"? Well, words do hurt, but throwing insults back at prejudiced people lowers you to their level. Words can also be powerful tools for change. Read and become informed. Think about what you learn and of positive ways you can use it. Reply to negative

comments with respect. You'll not only keep your dignity, but you'll also feel better about it while making your point. For example, if someone calls you a whale, you can say, "Aren't they the most interesting animals? Did you know they also have hearts the size of a sports car?"

4. **Speak up.** Don't hide your feelings. Talk about weight discrimination when you see or experience it. Let everyone know how hurtful it is, not only to you but to society as a whole. Bringing the problem into the open not only informs people, but it also makes you feel stronger and better able to cope.

5. **Decide to be happy.** Tell your family and friends that you have decided to accept the way you are. Ask them to work on accepting you, too.

6. **Take action.** Don't buy products from companies that are not respectful of others' sizes or that seek only to make money from people's issues with weight. Let the companies know how you feel about their ads.

7. **Help others.** Thinking of ways to help others can make you think less about your problems. Send cards, write encouraging notes, or make a gift for someone who needs a lift.

8. **Ban fat jokes.** If someone tells a fat joke, don't laugh at it to fit in. Tell the others you don't think it's funny. Refuse to watch television shows or movies or listen to radio programs that tell them.

9. **Be aware of media messages.** Question material you read and see in magazines, in books, in newspapers, on Web sites, and in other media sources. If they

present fat-biased material, let others know. Blog about it. E-mail customer service departments and let them know what they are saying could make others feel bad.

10. **Stand up for each other.** If you witness discrimination, stand up for the victim. Tell those who are doing it that it isn't right. Complain loudly until they stop. Refuse to back down. If it happens at school, report it to a teacher, counselor, or administrator you trust. If no one does anything about it, tell your parents, a religious leader, or another outside authority. Let your school or community newspaper know about it, too.

11. **Do what you can to help.** Join groups to fight against weight discrimination. Write letters to leaders about changing discrimination laws to include size. Refuse to buy products from companies who use only thin models. Write or e-mail customer service departments and tell them why.

12. **Get to know people of all sizes and shapes.** Respect others for who they are, not for what they look like. Remember that every human being is worthy of friendship and love.

13. **Lead changes.** If a time comes for you to choose partners or teams, pick someone whom you think might be left out. Or, volunteer to draw numbers or names so that everyone gets an equal chance.

14. **Ask for help.** Health professionals and counselors are trained to help you feel better about things that bother you, including your weight or how people treat you because of it. Thinking of some questions to ask

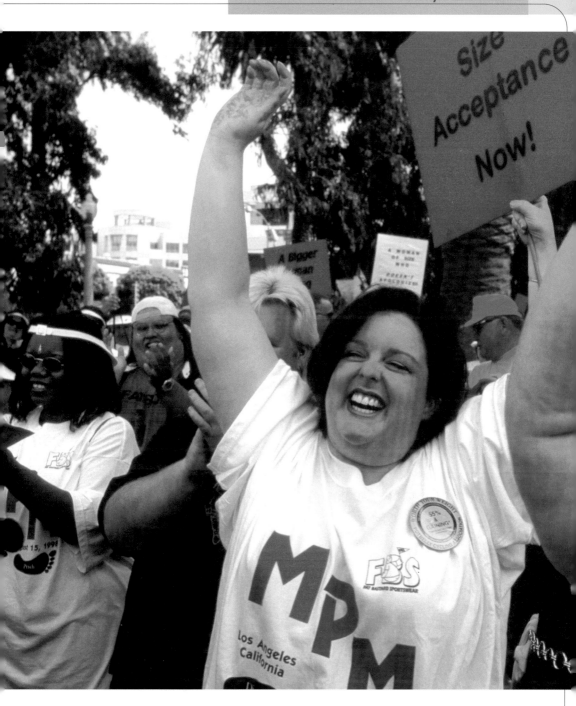

It takes work to change people's ways of thinking. Taking part in public rallies, letter-writing campaigns, and boycotts are all ways to end obesity discrimination.

51

beforehand gives you something to lean on when you go to them for help.

It is important to remember that people have hidden biases against certain differences. That includes doctors and nurses. But that is their problem, not yours. If you feel your doctor or counselor isn't listening to you or is focusing more on your weight than on you as a person, speak up. Ask them to explain their comments if you don't understand. Let them know if they make you feel uncomfortable. If you feel unhappy with the care they've given you, tell your parents, guardian, or a trusted adult. Ask them for help in finding a different doctor or counselor. You deserve to find someone who is willing to listen.

TEN GREAT QUESTIONS TO ASK A DOCTOR

1. My family nags me about my weight. How can I make them stop?
2. Is a diet the best way to control my weight?
3. If I lose weight, will people stop teasing me?
4. I exercise and eat right, but I'm still heavier than anyone I see on television. How can I look like them?
5. A teacher told my mom I'm obese. Does that mean I'm going to die soon?
6. Why am I short and fat, but my older brother is tall and skinny?
7. My best friend always complains about her weight and tells me how fat she is. It makes me feel bad because I'm a lot bigger than she is. What should I do?

8. The physical education teacher always makes my overweight friend run extra laps. Is that harmful?

9. Why do guys seem to just like skinny girls?

10. What can I do to stop hating my body?

WHAT NOW?

Facing discrimination can make you feel helpless and alone. But you don't have to sit by and let it happen. The National Association to Advance Fat Acceptance says, "We come in all sizes . . . understand it, support it, accept it."

Helen Keller was deaf and blind. She knew all about being helpless and alone before her teacher, Anne Sullivan, taught her the meaning of words. Keller went on to college and became a world-famous writer and speaker. She said, "The best and most beautiful things in the world cannot be seen or even touched—they must be felt with the heart."

We need to look within people, beyond our different shapes and sizes, to see who we truly are. We bring our similarities to the party. But it's our differences that give us reasons to celebrate.

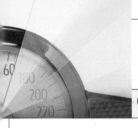

Glossary

ancestors The people or group from which you are descended.

anorexia A serious eating disorder that causes people, especially teenage girls, to starve themselves for fear of weight gain.

body mass index (BMI) A government-approved measure of body fat based on a person's height and weight.

bulimia A serious eating disorder that involves compulsive overeating that is usually followed by intentional vomiting or laxative abuse.

calorie A measurement of energy derived from food.

depression A mental disorder in which a person is sad and inactive and has low self-esteem.

environment The social and cultural conditions that influence the life of a person or human community.

gene A part of a cell that contains chemical information that controls inherited body traits or activity.

heredity The passing on of genes and genetic traits from parent to offspring.

obese A condition of having too much body fat defined as having a score of more than 30 on the body mass index.

overweight A condition of having more than average weight when compared to height or a score of 25 to 29.9 on the body mass index.

plague A disastrous evil or a cause for great discomfort and unhappiness.

ridicule The act of making fun of someone or something.

scapegoat A person or thing taking the blame for others.

sibling One of two or more individuals having the same parents or sometimes only one parent in common.

strategy The art of making or employing plans or tricks to achieve a goal.

suicide The act of killing oneself on purpose.

thyroid A large endocrine gland at the base of the neck that produces hormones that affect growth, development, and metabolism.

toxic A description of something caused by a poison or another harmful agent.

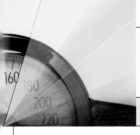

For More Information

Center for Screen-Time Awareness
1200 29th Street NW
Lower Level #1
Washington, DC 20007
(202) 333-9220
Web site: http://www.tvturnoff.org
This site offers facts, research, and support for those who wish
to decrease television time.

MyPyramid.gov
Center for Nutrition Policy and Promotion
U.S. Department of Agriculture
3101 Park Center Drive, Room 1034
Alexandria, VA 22302-1594
(888) 779-7264
Web site: http://www.mypyramid.gov
Information about exercise and healthy eating are available at
this Web site, as well as a tracking function that allows for
measuring food intake.

National Association to Advance Fat Acceptance (NAAFA)
P.O. Box 22510
Oakland, CA 94609
(916) 558-6880
Web site: http://www.naafa.org

This group works to improve the lives of fat people and get rid of discrimination based on body size.

Obesity Action Coalition
4511 North Himes Avenue, Suite 250
Tampa, FL 33614
(800) 717-3117
Web site: http://www.obesityaction.org
This organization is dedicated to educating and helping those affected by obesity, morbid obesity, and childhood obesity.

Rudd Center for Food Policy and Obesity
Yale University
309 Edwards Street
New Haven, CT 06520
(203) 432-6700
Web site: http://www.yaleruddcenter.org
This site provides information about the center's work to improve the world's diet, prevent obesity, and reduce weight stigma.

Web Sites

Due to the changing nature of Internet links, Rosen Publishing has developed an online list of Web sites related to the subject of this book. This site is updated regularly. Please use this link to access the list:

http://www.rosenlinks.com/uno/obdi

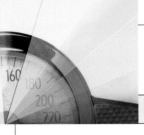

For Further Reading

Bennett, Cheri. *Life in the Fat Lane*. New York, NY: Delacorte Press, 1998.

Gay, Kathlyn. *Am I Fat? The Obesity Issue for Teens*. Berkeley Heights, NJ: Enslow Publishers, 2006.

Holt, Kimberly Willis. *When Zachary Beaver Comes to Town*. New York, NY: Henry Holt, 1999.

Kirberger, Kimberly. *No Body's Perfect*. New York, NY: Scholastic, 2003.

Mackler, Carolyn. *The Earth, My Butt and Other Big Round Things*. London, UK: Walker Books, Ltd., 2006.

Schlosser, Eric, and Charles Wilson. *Chew on This*. New York, NY: Houghton Mifflin, 2006.

Youth Communication. *I Took Dieting Too Far: Teens Write About Obesity and Body Image*. New York, NY: Youth Communication/NY Center, 2005.

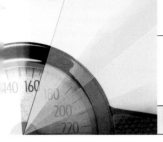

Bibliography

ABC News. "Tyra Banks Experiences Obesity Through Fat Suit." November 2005. Retrieved November 2007 (http://abcnews.go.com/GMA/story?id=1280787).

Ackman, Dan. "The Case of the Fat Aerobic Instructor." *Forbes*, May 2002. Retrieved September 2007 (http://www.forbes.com/people/2002/05/09/0509portnick.html).

American Obesity Association. "My Story." May 2005. Retrieved November 3, 2007 (http://obesity1.tempdomainname.com/subs/story/entirestory.shtml).

Aronson, David. "Best of: No Laughing Matter." *Teaching Tolerance*, Fall 1997. Retrieved October 2007 (http://www.tolerance.org/teach/magazine/features.jsp?p=0&is=35&ar=515).

Cromie, William J. "Gene Defect Found to Cause Obesity." *Harvard University Gazette*, October 1998. Retrieved October 2007 (http://www.hno.harvard.edu/gazette/1998/10.01/GeneDefectFound.html).

Crute, Sheree. "Growing Pains." *NEA Today*, March 2005. Retrieved September 8, 2007 (http://www.nea.org/neatoday/0503/coverstory.html).

Freydkin, Donna. "Stars Carry Curves with Confidence." *USA Today*, February 2007. Retrieved November 3, 2007 (http://www.usatoday.com/life/people/2007-02-18-curvy-celebs_x.htm?loc=interstitialskip).

Gaesser, Glenn A., Ph.D. "Death by Adipose? The Fuzzy Logic and Fuzzy Math of the Latest 'Obesity Kills' Statistic." *Health at Every Size Journal*, Vol. 18, No. 3, July/August 2004.

Jackson, Camille. "Fat . . . So?" *Teaching Tolerance*. Retrieved November 2007 (http://www.tolerance.org/teach/magazine/features.jsp?is=40&ar=779&pa=5).

Loewry, Michael. "Working with Fat Children in Schools." *Radiance*, Fall 1998. Retrieved October 2007 (http://www.radiancemagazine.com/kids_project/working.htm).

National Association to Advance Fat Acceptance. "Stop Targeting the Kids." January 2007. Retrieved October 2007 (http://www.naafa.org/newevents/kids.html).

National Center for Health Statistics. "Obesity Still a Major Problem." 2006. Retrieved August 28, 2007 (http://www.cdc.gov/nchs/pressroom/06facts/obesity03_04.htm).

Nelson, Blythe. "Just Fat, Not Stupid." *Radiance*, Spring 1999. Retrieved October 2007 (http://www.radiancemagazine.com/issues/1999/spring_99/spring99_teen_scene.htm).

Obesity Action Coalition. *Understanding Obesity, Understanding Obesity Stigma, Understanding Childhood Obesity*. Retrieved December 11, 2007 (http://www.obesityaction.org/resources/brochures-guides.php).

Offutt, Susan, and Craig Gundersen. "Farm Poverty Lowest in U.S. History." *Amber Waves*, September 2005. Retrieved September 2007 (http://www.ers.usda.gov/AmberWaves/September05/Features/FarmPoverty.htm).

Patterson, Amanda. "Growing Up Fat." *Radiance*, Winter 1996. Retrieved October 2007 (http://www.radiancemagazine.com/issues/1996/winter96_apatterson.html).

Puhl, Rebecca, Ph.D. "Childhood Obesity and Stigma." *Childhood Obesity*. Retrieved October 2007 (http://www.obesityaction.org/resources/oacnews/oacnews7/Childhood%20Obesity%20and%20Stigma.pdf).

Rubel, Jean, Ph.D. *Radiance*, Fall 1987. Retrieved October 2007 (http://www.radiancemagazine.com/kids_project/when_children_hate.html).

Shanker, Wendy. "Q&A with Wendy Shanker." Wendy's World. Retrieved November 2007 (http://www.wendyshanker.com/meet_qa.html).

Silverman, Stephen M. "Chewing the Fat with Gwyneth Paltrow." *People*, November 2001. Retrieved October 2007 (http://www.people.com/people/article/0,,622921,00.html).

Weight-Control Information Network. "Statistics Related to Overweight and Obesity." Retrieved October 2007 (http://win.niddk.nih.gov/statistics/index.htm).

Williams, Carla. "Eating Healthy Might Prove Too Expensive for Poor." ABC News, November 2007. Retrieved November 2007 (http://abcnews.go.com/Health/Diet/story?id=3807128&page=1).

Williams, Dana. "Making Room for Size Acceptance." *Parenting for Tolerance*, August 2002. Retrieved October 2007 (http://www.tolerance.org/parents/kidsarticle.jsp?p=0&ar=1).

Wysocki, Kristen. "Barbie: Attainable Beauty or Impossible Perfection?" Retrieved November 2007 (http://people.bu.edu/kwysocki).

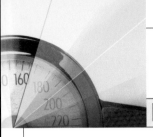

Index

About the Author

Dale-Marie Bryan writes for all shapes and sizes of children and adults as a curriculum specialist in southeast Kansas. She first experienced obesity discrimination in elementary school.

Photo Credits

Editor: Nicholas Croce

29.25

4/14/10

LONGWOOD PUBLIC LIBRARY
800 Middle Country Road
Middle Island, NY 11953
(631) 924-6400
mylpl.net

LIBRARY HOURS

Monday-Friday	9:30 a.m. - 9:00 p.m.
Saturday	9:30 a.m. - 5:00 p.m.
Sunday (Sept-June)	1:00 p.m. - 5:00 p.m.